Angels & Monsters

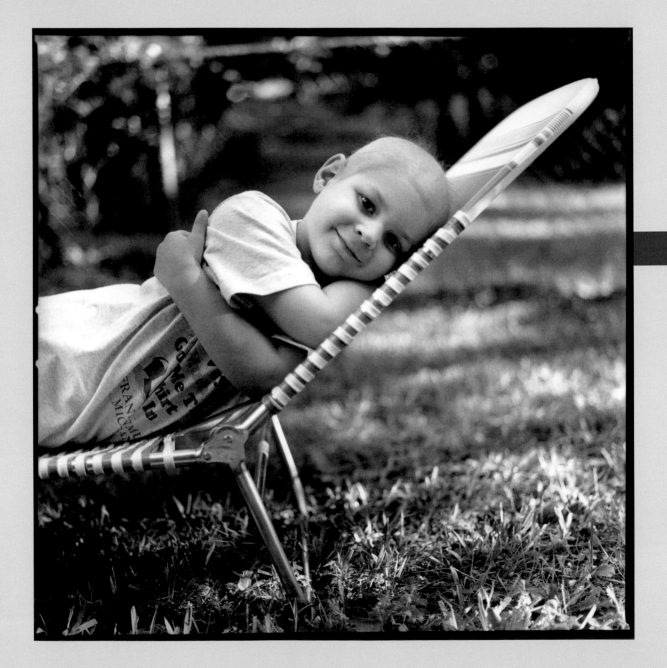

Angels &
Monsters

A child's eye view of cancer

ART THERAPY
Lisa Murray

PHOTOGRAPHY
Billy Howard

★

Foreword
Jeff Foxworthy

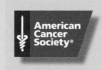

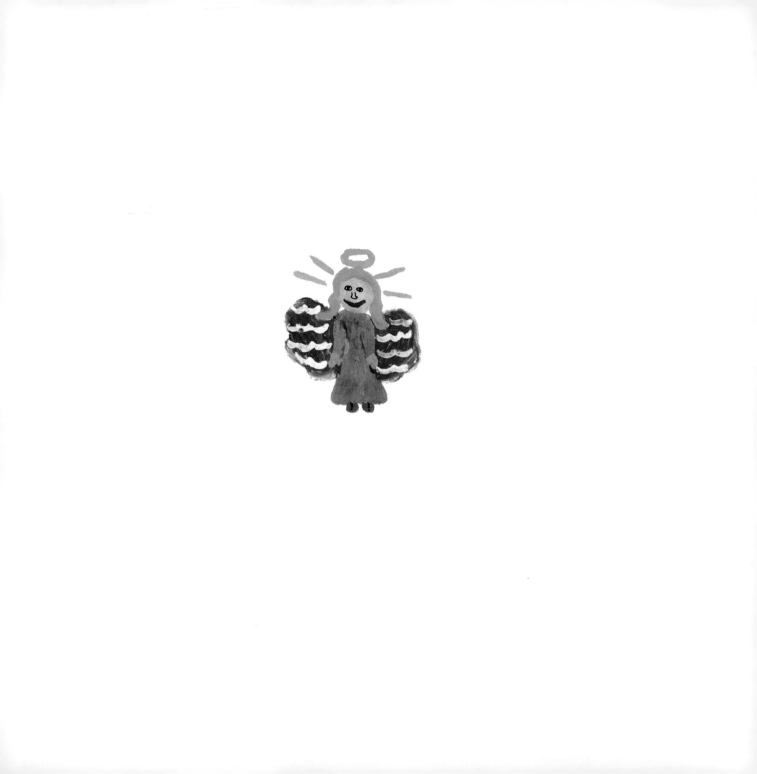

Angels & Monsters
honors the twenty-five courageous children
whose gifts to us are found in its pages.

The book is dedicated to those we hold in loving memory

Elizabeth Kate Cleveland
Victoria Grace Fowler
David Loyd Harris, Jr.
Ian Galloway Horner
Jacob Cicero Hulsey
James Coleman Lee
Courtney Yvonne Rush
David Louis Tardif

Published by
American Cancer Society • Health Content Products
1599 Clifton Road NE • Atlanta, Georgia 30329, USA
800-ACS-2345 • www.cancer.org

The concept for this book grew out of the art exhibition "Godzilla® vs. Cancer," directed by Lisa Murray and Billy Howard, and first shown in June 1994 at Marcia Wood Gallery in Atlanta.

Godzilla® & ©2002 Toho Co., Ltd. All rights reserved. Used courtesy of Toho Co., Ltd.

Printed in Spain

5   4   3   2   1   02   03   04   05   06

LIBRARY OF CONGRESS CATALOGING-IN-PUBLICATION DATA

Murray, Lisa.
   Angels and monsters : a child's eye view of cancer / art therapy by Lisa Murray ; photography by Billy Howard.
      p. ; cm.
   ISBN 0-944235-22-0 (alk. paper)
   1. Cancer in children--United States. 2. Arts--Therapeutic use. 3. Children's art--United States. 4. Cancer in children--United States--Portraits.
   [DNLM: 1. Art Therapy--Adolescence--United States--Drawings. 2. Art Therapy--Adolescence--United States--Personal Narratives. 3. Art Therapy--Adolescence--United States--Portraits. 4. Art Therapy--Child--United States--Drawings. 5. Art Therapy--Child--United States--Personal Narratives. 6. Art Therapy--Child--United States--Portraits. 7. Neoplasms--psychology --Adolescence--United States--Drawings. 8. Neoplasms--psychology--Adolescence--United States--Personal Narratives. 9. Neoplasms--psychology--Adolescence--United States--Portraits. 10. Neoplasms--psychology--Child--United States--Drawings. 11. Neoplasms--psychology--Child--United States--Personal Narratives. 12. Neoplasms--psychology--Child--United States--Portraits. 13. Longitudinal Studies--United States--Drawings. 14. Longitudinal Studies--United States--Personal Narratives. 15. Longitudinal Studies--United States--Portraits. QZ 275 M982a 2002] I. Howard, Billy. II. American Cancer Society. III. Title.
   RC281.C4 M875 2002
   618.92'994065156--dc21

                                                                                    2002005828

Text written by
Beth Dawkins Bassett

*Book and jacket design
and production by*
Shock Design, Inc.

Managing Editor
Beth Dawkins Bassett

American Cancer Society
HEALTH CONTENT PRODUCTS

Diane Scott-Lichter
Director, Publishing Strategy

Candace J. Magee
Book Publishing Manager

Terri Ades, MS, APRN-BC, AOCN
Editorial Review

Title page and cover photo: Jacob, age 5

Table of
Contents

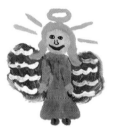

Old souls in little bodies

Spend some time in the presence of children with cancer, and you're never quite the same again. I've met famous actors, singers, athletes, even a few presidents, and none were as remarkable as these children.

I can't tell you the exact moment it happened, but through my work with children with cancer, I went from avoiding to embracing these children. I've laughed with them, cried for them, and delivered eulogies in their honor. Working with them has been one of the greatest blessings of my life.

Physically and mentally, these children have been to places you don't ever want to visit. They have stood at the edge and stared into the dark void. Yet they have a depth, dignity, and spirit I've never seen anywhere else. I've often said God gives them something extra, and they use it.

The wisdom of the ages tells us to live each day as if it were our last. Sadly, most of us fall short, but these kids do just that. They are able to milk every bit of joy and irony out of every moment. They are old souls in little bodies.

They will tell you that they just want to be normal. They are anything but. Having stood toe to toe with this monster, cancer, they are never the same again, and having known them, neither am I.

—Jeff Foxworthy

From the art therapist

These are children I worked with. They and others like them are my inspiration. My sole desire for doing this book is to let people know that these children have something very important to say. It is their gift to us if we are wise enough to pause and accept it.

The feelings these children express run the gamut from anger and despair to pride and strength. Some shout, others whisper. All reach for hope along the road to remission with the goal of eventually referring to themselves as survivors.

These children offer a unique and intimate look into their souls. They were asked to draw the thing that threatened to steal away their lives. They responded with uninhibited, forthright images and then added to that their own words. Photographs complete the expression by showing us who they are.

While this book honors all these children, it is for me offered especially in memory of Katie Cleveland, Grace Fowler, and David Tardif, who died before their art work was first shown in June 1994. Both Katie and David knew they were going to die when I asked them to participate. Both expressed a desire—a need—to make and leave their mark. I am thankful I could help them. It is a humbling experience.

As we prepared this book, it was my task to contact the families of the twenty-five children in its pages. Reminiscing with them was an uplifting experience. Many of the children I had known are adults now, some with children of their own. The families of the children who did not survive their illness remember their courage and love and the good times they shared. All the memories came flooding back. I remembered in particular the day I took my then-newborn son to see David Tardif. David held him and said, "I want one of these." "And I want him to be like you," I responded. David smiled and said, "All but the cancer."

—*Lisa Murray*

From the photographer

These children are at war.

Their weapons are grace, courage, and spirits that defy the insidious disease they fight—cancer.

At a time in their lives when they should be exploring a world full of infinite possibilities, they face a finite possibility, yet they show a richness and focus that sets them apart as they take from still moments understanding that may escape the rest of us.

But they have left clues.

At age seventeen, David T. sees in small, colored glass beads a universe in harmony.

Tonkya, age eighteen, shows us the turmoil and depth of her mind through shapes and words all painted in the vivid colors she loves and hopes will cheer others.

Eric L., age eleven, has risen from a vortex of hopelessness to become an intense, introspective young man with a passionate artistic voice.

Each of the twenty-five children in these pages has explored his or her overwhelming reality and given us a message both innocent and profound.

Many have found a path—through imagination—to a wisdom that confronts our greatest fears with charity, humor, and affection.

Each has in his or her soul the essence of truth—pure, honest, and undiluted by adulthood. Their truth has no room for negotiation. It is simple and infinite, and it is their gift to us.

—Billy Howard

Children at war with cancer

IN THE WORLD OF FIVE-YEAR-OLD JARED'S BUSY IMAGINATION, the movie monster Godzilla®
was a main character, a splendid, tremendously strong, omnipresent fellow
roaming the planet, seeking out and destroying evil in scenario after scenario. The
boy spent many pleasant hours watching the monster on film, playing with Godzilla®
action figures, and sometimes pretending he *was* Godzilla®.

But something went wrong in the happy-go-lucky boy's life that year he was
five. His parents noticed he did not seem to feel well, didn't react to events in his
characteristic way. They took him to a pediatrician, who found that Jared had a
tumor. Subsequent tests showed the tumor was Burkitt's lymphoma, a fast-growing
form of cancer, but one for which treatment usually is effective. He was admitted to
a children's hospital for large initial doses of chemotherapy.

Art therapist Lisa Murray, who worked in the hospital, met Jared soon after he
entered. The strange sights and sounds and the big, cold machines in the boy's new
surroundings had frightened him, and she was called in to help. She brought a toy
alligator with her and played with him until he relaxed.

Some time later, when he had recovered in part from the first chemotherapy,
Murray asked Jared to use an art medium to show what he thought about having cancer.
She watched as he chose brightly colored markers from her array of media, then drew
a multi-storied purple hospital with many windows and a large door. Beside the hospital
he placed his spiny-backed old friend Godzilla®, standing as high as the building and
breathing red fire. Godzilla® was at work on yet another dangerous errand against evil.
He was destroying cancer.

In the language of art therapists, the drawing was age appropriate. Jared had
used the bright colors five year olds typically like and had drawn a favorite subject for
children his age—a super-hero. The drawing revealed other things, too. The many

windows and large door of the hospital indicated his own openness: he could freely receive and respond to the world around him. Further, his drawing was large enough to fill all the space on the page, an indication of self-confidence and strength. Murray detected some normal fear in the picture, but most of all it showed a classic conflict, a hero using his arsenal of weapons to battle a mighty foe. The body of this well-adjusted little boy had somehow been invaded by a powerful, mysterious presence, and he was prepared to fight it. Deep inside himself he had marshaled his strength.

For a number of years, Murray had looked on as seriously ill children like Jared expressed themselves in line and shape and color. They were naturally at home in the language of art and through it poured out the substance of their deepest thoughts. The more Murray watched the phenomenon, the more convinced she became that other people needed to see what she was seeing. These children needed a larger forum.

Without knowing it, Murray and photographer Billy Howard had reached parallel conclusions. Howard had been coming to the hospital for years, photographing the children for various publications and talking to them. He was, in fact, drawn to them. "They were going through so much," he said. "The treatment was painful, and they were losing their hair. They saw how their parents were suffering. And yet, they developed a kind of philosophical wisdom. They touched my soul." He decided that at some point he would compile a collection of the children's portraits.

Murray had seen Howard at the hospital, and although she did not know about his plans to compile a group of pictures, she approached him with an idea: she would like to show the children's art paired with their portraits. "I could see the light bulbs go off in his head," she said. "I could see his wheels turning." They agreed to begin the project.

After months of work, Murray and Howard opened an exhibition in June 1994 in an Atlanta art gallery. They called it "Godzilla® vs. Cancer." That exhibition became the basis for the book *Angels & Monsters*.

★

When Jared was diagnosed with cancer, he became one among the million-and-a-quarter people found to have the disease every year in the Unites States, and one among the subset of some 9,000 children under age fifteen. The diagnosis changes lives. Plans are put on hold, and days revolve around tests, rounds of treatment, and the central unknown: Will this person survive? Today, the statistical answer to that question is yes. More people diagnosed with cancer will survive than will die. We are, in fact, experiencing the first sustained decline in the overall death rate from cancer since record keeping began in the 1930s. Most types of the disease are now curable if found at an early stage, and some types are curable even if the cancer has spread. A cure for all cancers probably will not be seen for many years, but ways to slow the progress of the disease and treatments to prolong and improve the quality of life of people with cancer are continually emerging.

Although all the diseases we call cancer involve unchecked growth of abnormal cells, the causes, symptoms, means of diagnosis, and treatment of various types vary widely. Childhood cancer as a group differs from adult cancer in several important ways, including cause and the types of cancer that occur most frequently. In children, leukemias, nervous system tumors, lymph node cancers, bone cancers, soft tissue sarcomas, kidney cancers, eye cancers, and adrenal gland cancers are most often seen, while in adults, skin, prostate, breast, lung, and colorectal cancers lead the list.

Some forms of childhood cancer are the result of a familial predisposition, and in others, radiation exposure is a contributing factor. None are closely related to the lifestyle risk factors responsible for many adult forms. The cause of most childhood cancer is unknown.

Years ago, childhood cancer was almost always fatal, but the mortality rate has declined 50 percent since 1973. Seventy-seven percent of children diagnosed in 2002 will survive five years or more, an increase of nearly 40 percent since the early 1960s.

★

After Murray and Howard decided to build an exhibition around the art of children grappling with cancer, Murray chose twenty-five children and young people for whom she thought such an experience would be cathartic. They ranged in age from thirteen months to eighteen years. She worked with each child or young person individually and with no time pressure, first asking them to choose a medium and express what it was like to have cancer. Then, once the artwork was done, she asked them to tell her about it, and as they spoke, she wrote their words verbatim.

Some expressed despair, and some expressed anger at lives interrupted. Some drew pictures of the treatment they were undergoing, and some depicted their desire to escape treatment. Some drew their weeping mothers. One of the adolescents created a string of blue, green, and white beads representing Earth's water, plant life, and all living creatures. Of the white beads, he said, "We need to remember how small we really are in the whole scope of things." Several of the children depicted their precocious realizations about the transcendent value of love for family and friends. Several drew pictures that spoke to deep-seated religious convictions.

Often appearing in the pictures were figures at the ends of two extremes—fearful ones and completely benign ones. Jared drew a fearful creature—his favorite movie monster—as an advocate, a deadly weapon in the fight against cancer. Another boy pictured cancer itself as a monster. He called it "The Leukemia Monster." Several girls drew angels, the embodiment of goodness, beauty, hope. It was as if cancer had coaxed from these children images at the far reaches of human thought. Angels and monsters.

As Murray assembled the art and commentary, Howard set out to photograph each child. "The picture-taking became a special moment in their lives," he said. "Everything else was negative. They were being poked, prodded, examined. And then something different happened. Someone wanted to come and take their pictures. They enjoyed it, and their parents enjoyed it. Someone was acknowledging what they were going through. I felt glad to be with them. These were special events for them at a time in their lives that was without specialness."

By the time the exhibition began, three of the original twenty-five children had

4

died: David T., Grace, and Katie. Grace had been three years old. When asked what her abstract painting meant, she had said, "It means I love you." Katie and David, fourteen and seventeen, had known they were dying, and they had wanted to leave something behind as proof that they had lived. They believed that inclusion in the art exhibition would be partial fulfillment of that wish. Katie had drawn her guardian angel, and David had made the string of beads representing Earth.

In the years since the 1994 exhibition, cancer has taken the lives of five more of the children, and seventeen have survived, a rate almost identical to the corresponding national statistic. Those children and young people who survive have returned to normalcy with a deepened appreciation for life.

Among the survivors is Marcus, now twenty-three. Eight years ago, fifteen-year-old Marcus, full of despair, drew "The Leukemia Monster." Today, he is a strapping, six-foot-tall young man who writes poetry and is enrolled in truck-driving school for big rigs. His classmates say he smiles all the time.

★

Shortly after "Godzilla® vs. Cancer" opened, Murray, Howard, and one child who participated in it were interviewed on the television show "Good Morning, America." The child was Jessica S., then eleven. For her artwork she had drawn a friendship necklace—really two necklaces, each strung with half a heart. When the halves are joined at their jagged edges, they form one perfect heart. "Friends are forever," she wrote.

Jessica was thrilled to be in New York and on national television. She was interviewed wearing a pretty blue-and-white outfit, and matching tights covered her one leg. The other leg had been amputated the year before. Jessica is now a cancer survivor and is enrolled in college, studying psychology.

At the beginning of the television broadcast, the exhibition participants were shown shouting the show's usual greeting: "Good Morning, America!" Howard remembers that when the greeting was pre-filmed in Atlanta, all the children shouted uniformly except unstoppable Jared, who, wishing to be heard individually, kept saying, "Good Morning, America-a-a-a-a!" in take after take.

One year after the exhibition, Jared, by then six years old and in remission, created a new super-hero he called "ChemoKid." ChemoKid, the boy said, had "found the formula to fight Cancella. It's in his hand. The formula kills Cancella. Cancella falls down and splats to the ground. . . . The ChemoKid is the winner." Jared has survived cancer and is now thirteen years old and in the eighth grade.

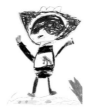

Through the pages of this book, you are invited to enter the world in which these children lived as they underwent treatment for cancer. It is a special world. No artifice exists there. The human spirit holds sway with complete honesty and great dignity. *Angels & Monsters* honors the lives of the children it portrays and the lives of other children like them everywhere.

The statistics given here come from *Cancer Facts & Figures 2002*. The author also is indebted to *Informed Decisions: The Complete Book of Cancer Diagnosis, Treatment, and Recovery, 2nd Edition,* by Eyre, Lange, and Morris. Both are publications of the American Cancer Society.

Opposite: Lisa Murray and Jacob, age 5

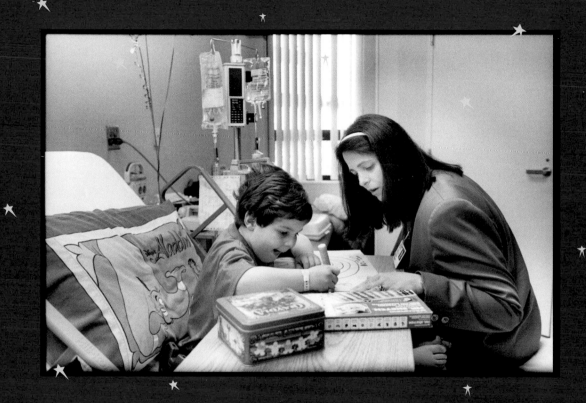

"*Take him and cut him out in little stars and
he will make the face of heaven so fine that
all the world will be in love with night.*"

SHAKESPEARE

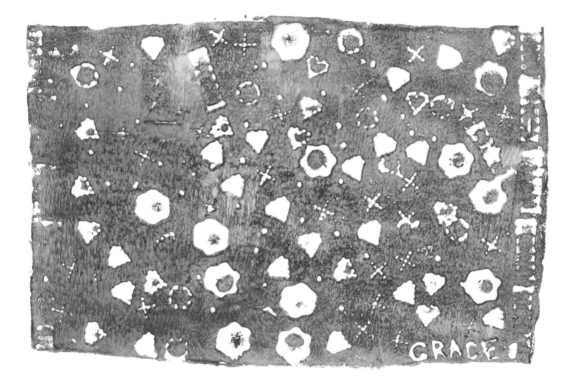

When Grace was asked what her picture said,
she replied: "It says I love you."

Grace
age 3

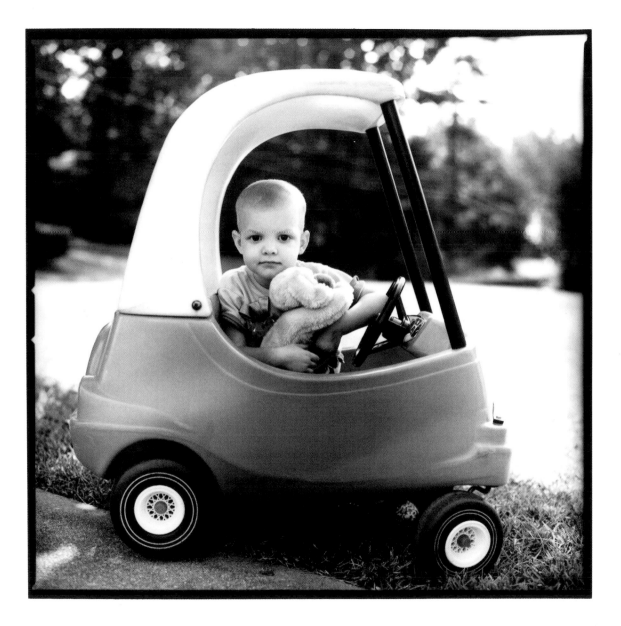

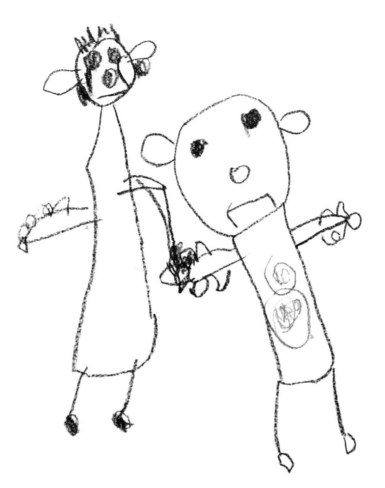

My mommy is crying because I have leukemia in my body.
My mommy is holding my hand. I feel sad because I have
leukemia in my body.

Artavius
age 6

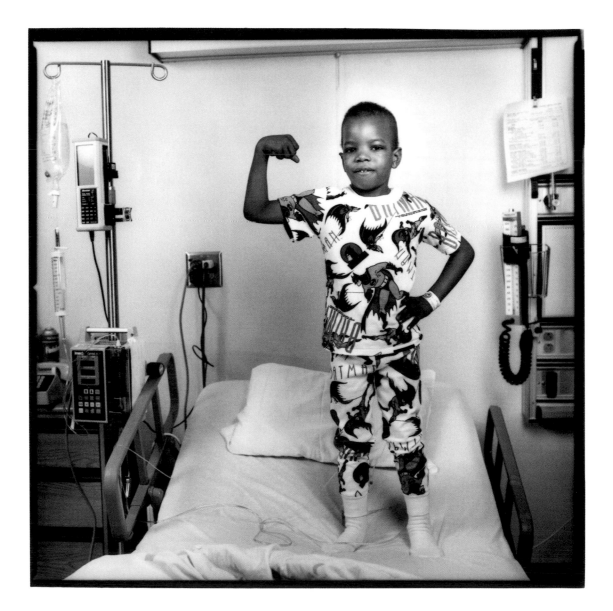

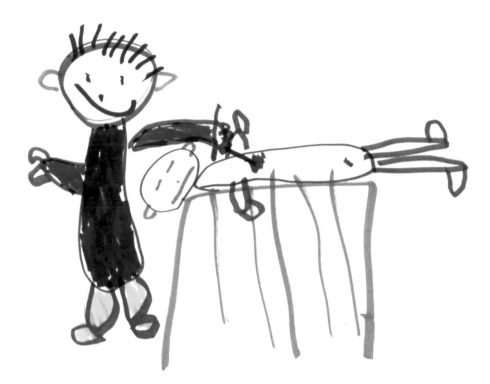

I'm getting a biopsy. The doctor just jabbed a little hole in my side. I had sleepy medicine. He was searching for leukemia. I have leukemia now but I still feel like a regular kid.

Jacob
age 5

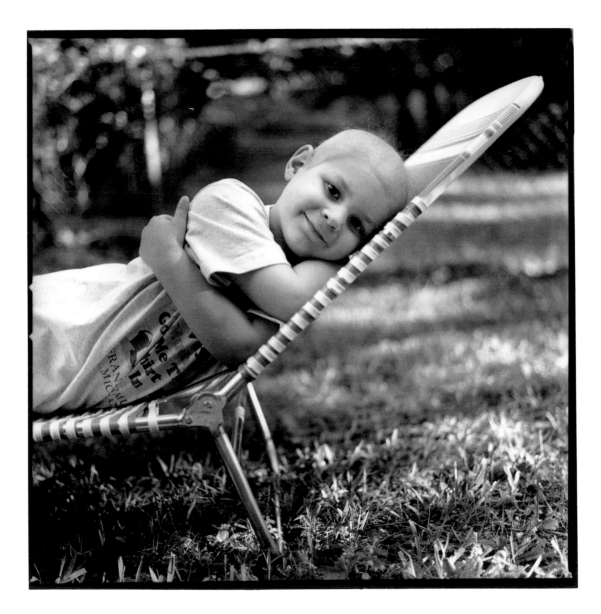

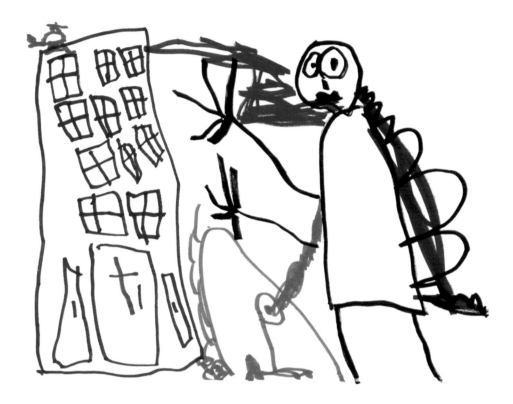

Godzilla® vs. the Hospital

Godzilla® is breathing fire on the hospital and is going to burn it down.
Godzilla® is going to win. The nurses can't stick him with their needles.
It wouldn't work because he'll growl and he'll get worser and worser.
He'll be mad. The doctors won't even get a chance to listen to his heart
with their stethoscope. Then Godzilla® goes back home to under the sea.

Jared
age 5

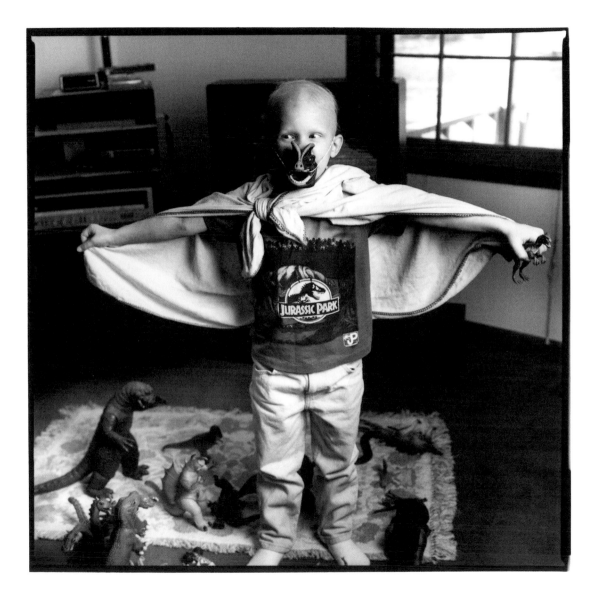

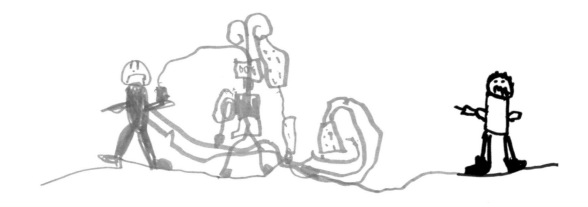

Seth

It made me sick and throw up. I wanted to go home!
My IV pumps made noise and kept me up at night.

Seth
age 8

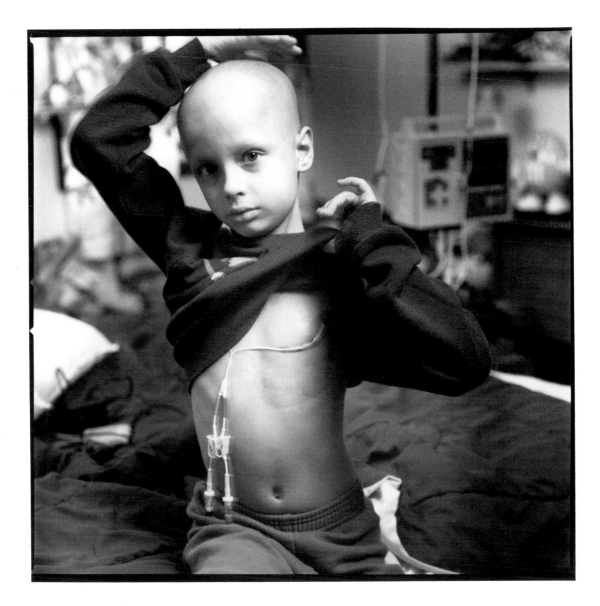

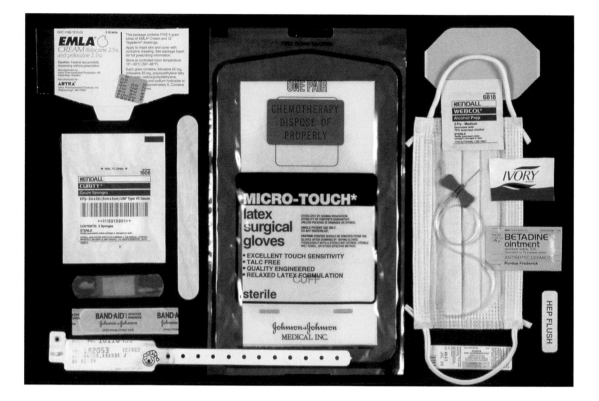

I'm sick of seeing this stuff.

Amanda
age 14

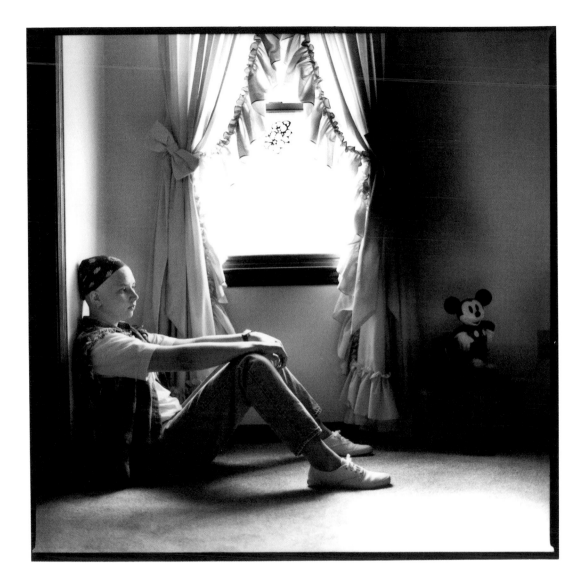

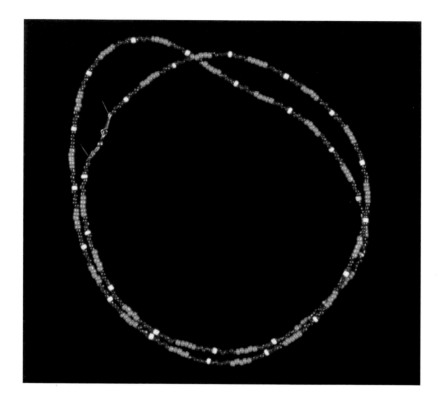

The necklace is mostly blue because our planet is mostly water,
then green for all plant life and finally the smallest...the white for
ALL living creatures, including human beings, because we need to
remember how small we really are in the whole scope of things.

David T.
age 17

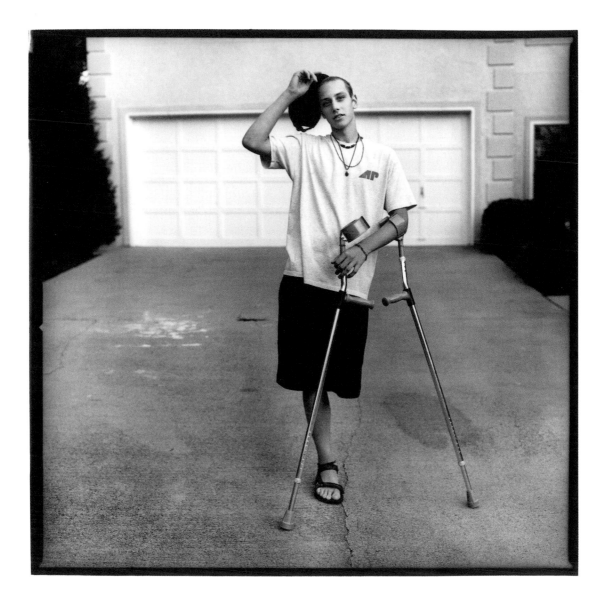

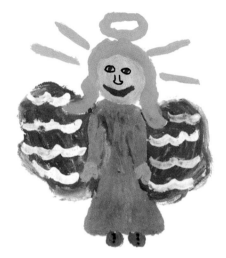

I believe that every child has a guardian Angel to watch over them. This is how my Angel looks.

Take heed that ye despise not one of these little ones;
for I say unto you, that in heaven their angels do always
behold the face of my Father which is in heaven.

MATTHEW 18:10

Katie
age 14

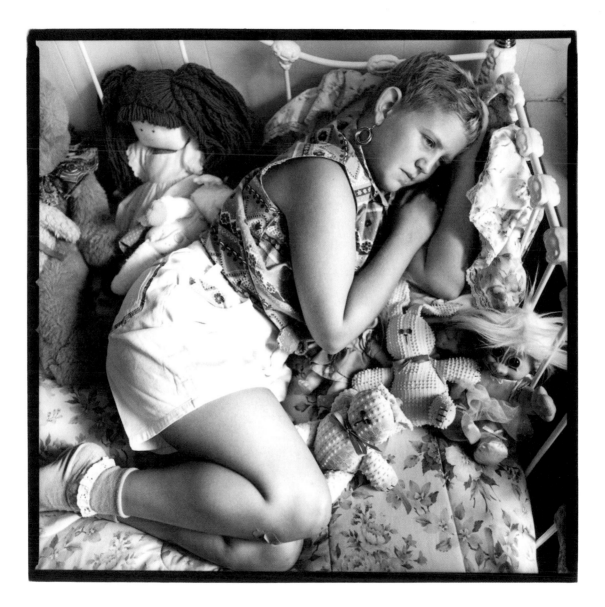

This is what I first thought was going to happen to me when I got cancer. I would die automatically. But now I'm half way through my treatments for this dreadful disease and I feel like I'm going to live. The thought of dying still scares me though. The name of this painting is… "Till Death Do Us Part."

Eric L.
age 11

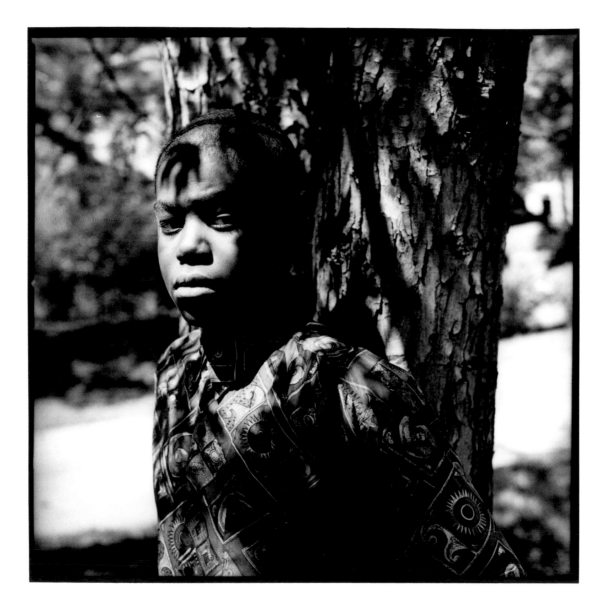

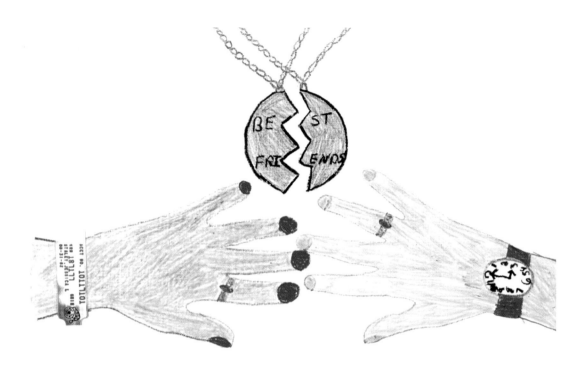

Sometimes I feel like this experience will never end. But I know it will. Having my friends makes me want to keep on going. Friends are forever.

Jessica S.
age 11

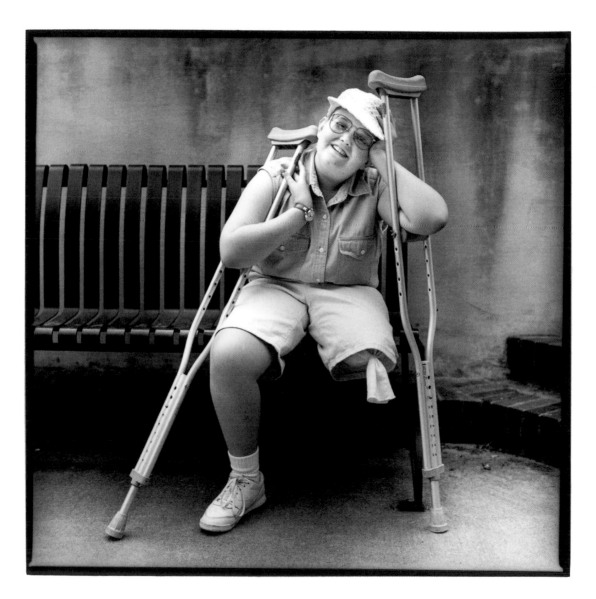

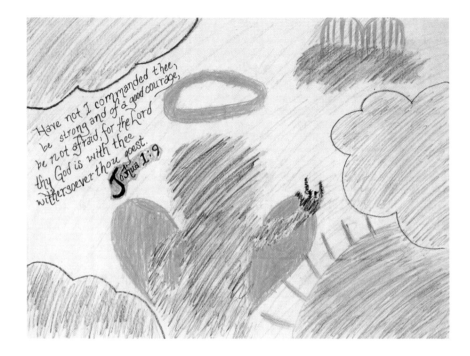

Just after my diagnosis, I had a "dream," more real than any dream before. I saw an angel, just the size of a small child, who smiled at me and then signed "I love you" in sign language. Next thing, I was standing at the gates of heaven where I was informed that I could not enter. It then occurred to me that perhaps I hadn't yet fulfilled all that God planned for me. Now, I always use my faith in God, as well as my dream, to carry me through everything.

Jennifer
age 18

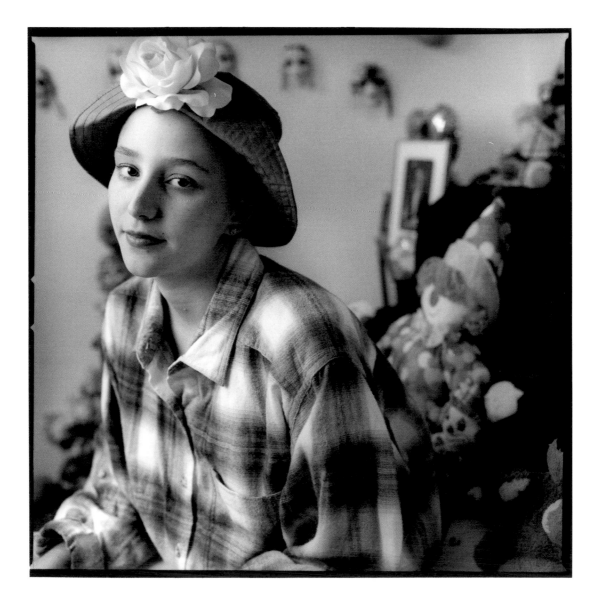

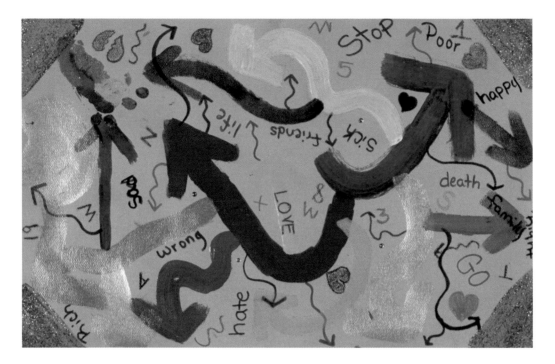

Confused Mind

A picture that shows my mind when it is confused. Plus it has so many different things on it. That keeps your mind occupied for a while.

I did the picture in different colors because I love a lot of colors. They usually cheer people up.

The arrows represent the many different ways my mind is thinking. The numbers represent the many children I know that have died of cancer.

Tonkya
age 18

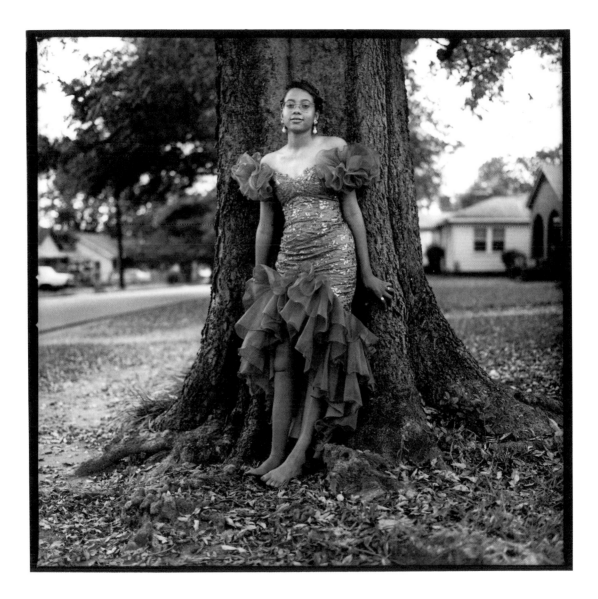

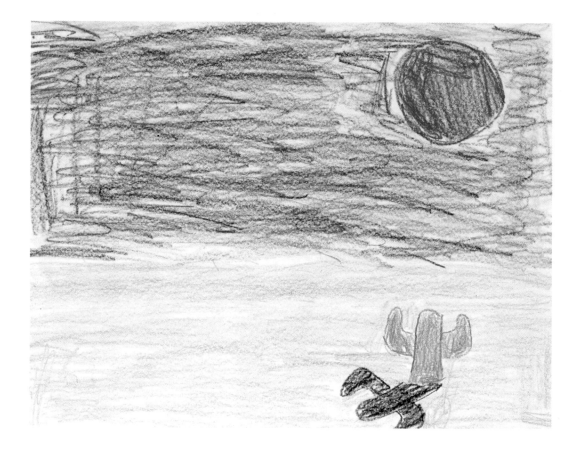

Having cancer is like being all alone and lost in the desert.

Jeremiah
age 13

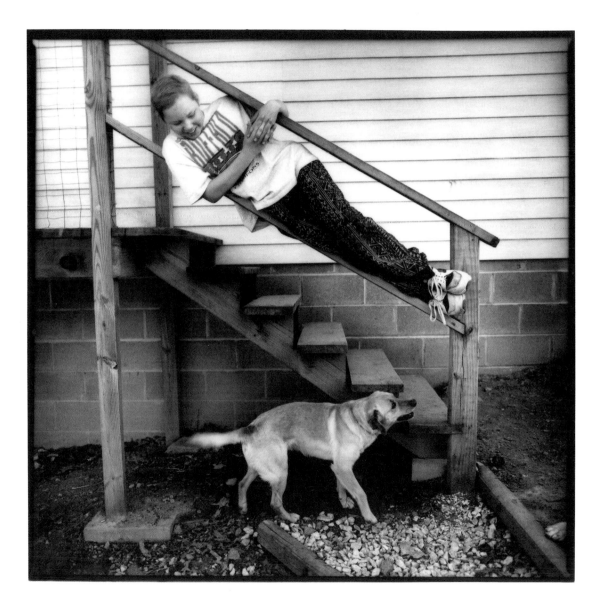

Never hold your head up high and think you've got it made, because by the time you look over your shoulder, it starts all over again!

Barbara
age 15

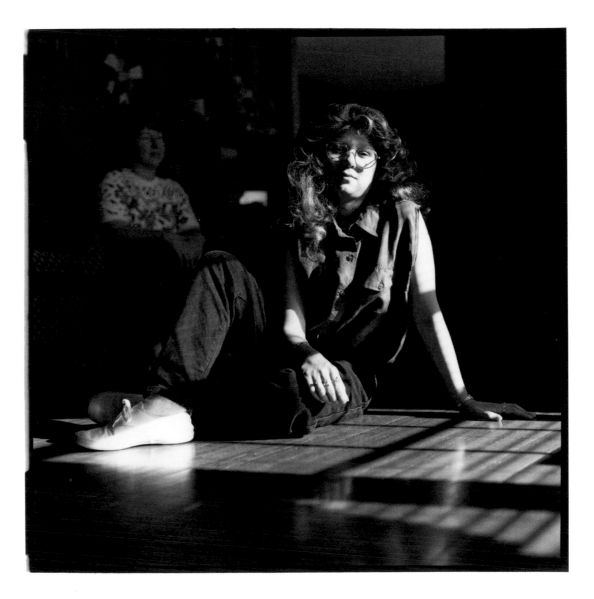

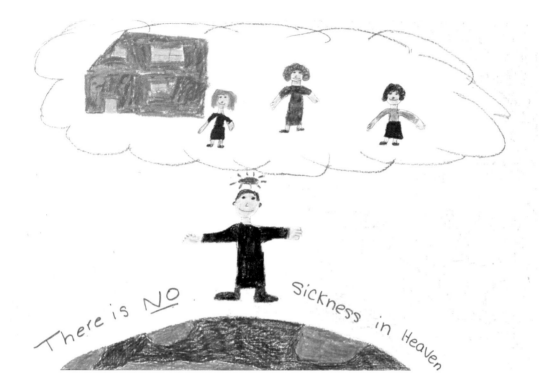

There is NO Sickness in Heaven

I never really felt angry when I got cancer. Three of my friends have gotten saved because of my experience. Maybe that wouldn't have happened if I hadn't gotten cancer.

Kelli
age 13

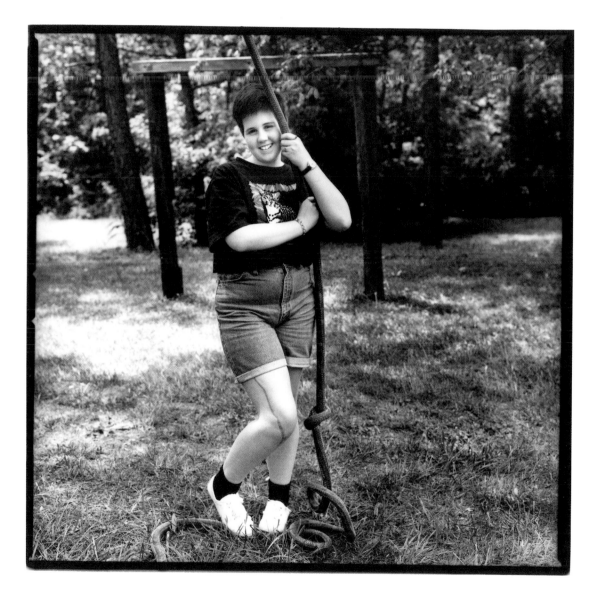

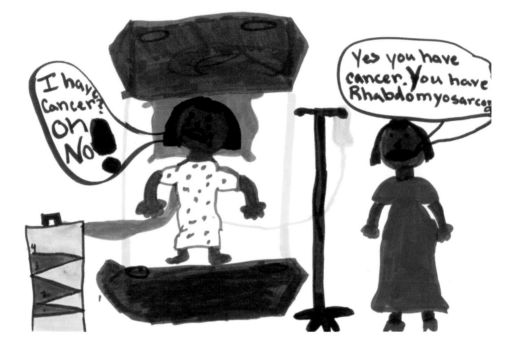

This is how I felt when they told me I had cancer. It was very scary. I cried when they told me my hair was going to fall out.

Courtney
age 9

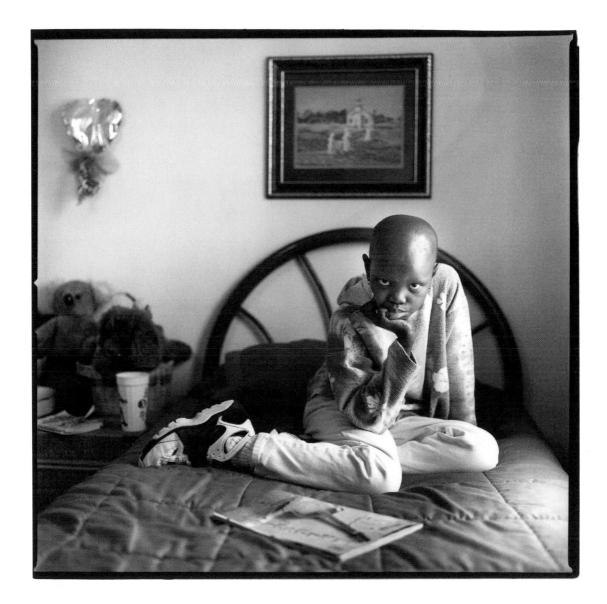

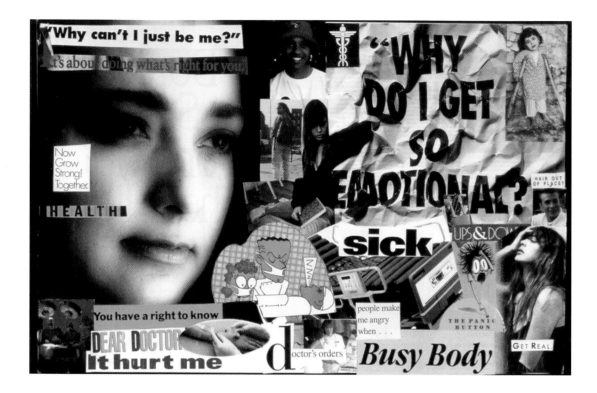

This is how I feel about what has happened to me.

Kimsy
age 14

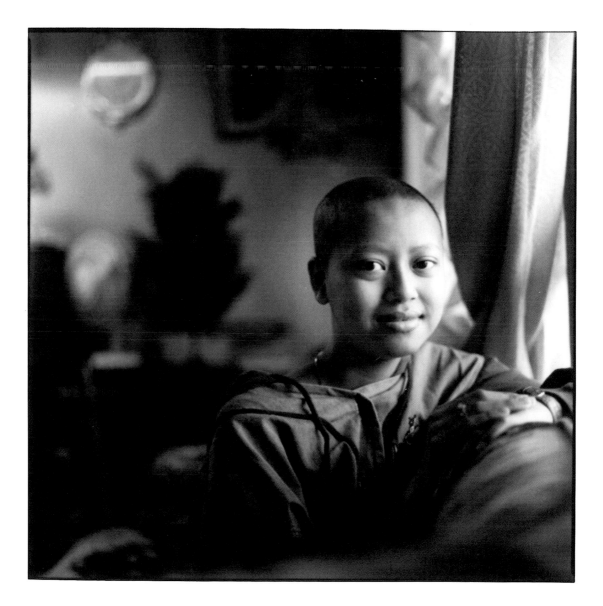

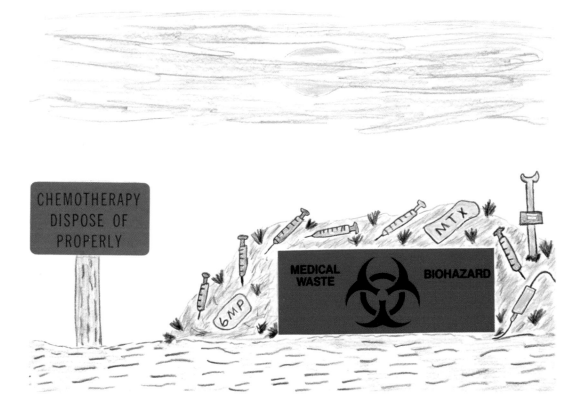

Having leukemia and dealing with chemotherapy is like one
big pile of dump full of anger, confusion, and pain.

James
age 16

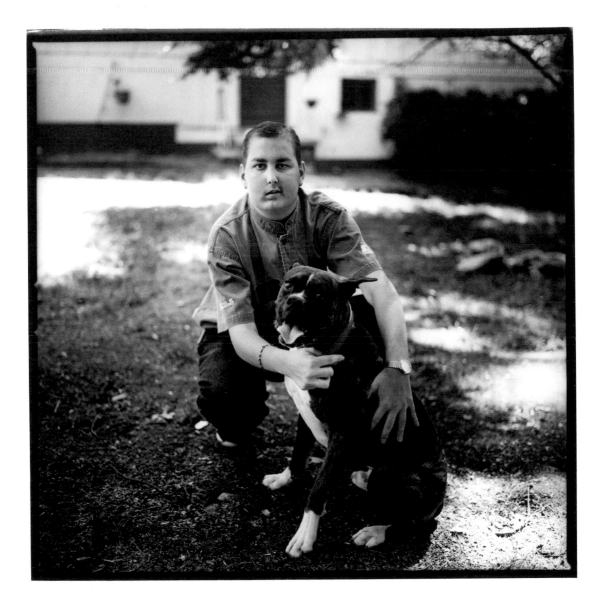

43

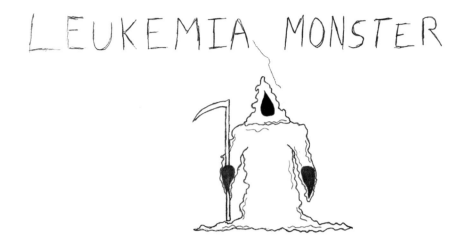

The Leukemia Monster — Death Becomes Me.

Marcus
age 15

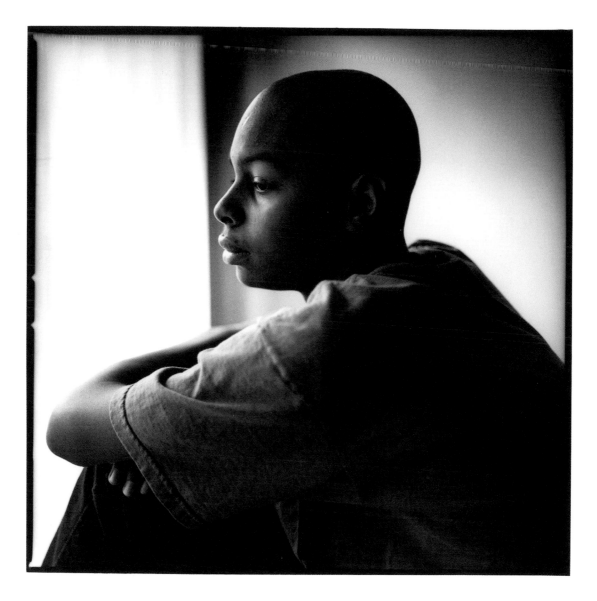

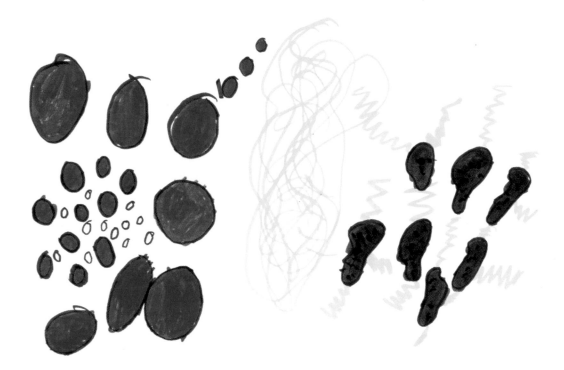

The yellow chemotherapy is going in my body to kill the bad
cancer cells so the normal cells can win. The chemotherapy is
like lightning and blasts the bad cancer cells. The platelets are the
biggest and the red cells are the middlest and the white cells are
the smallest. I'm getting by because the bad cancer cells are dying.

Jessica B.
age 7

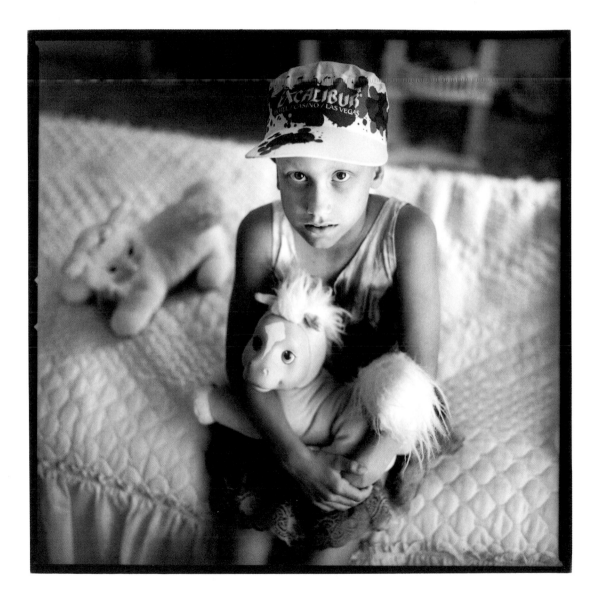

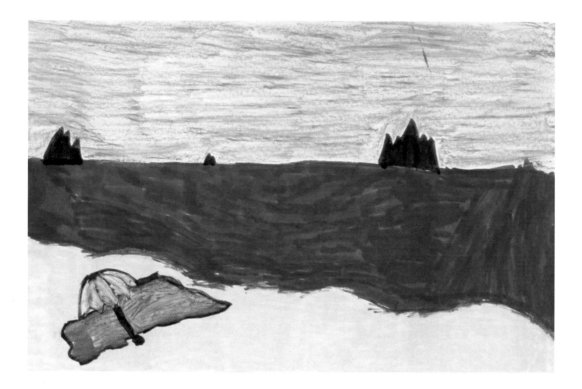

Sometimes I imagine myself on a vacation away from my tumor.
It helps me get away from my problems.

Eric D.
age 10

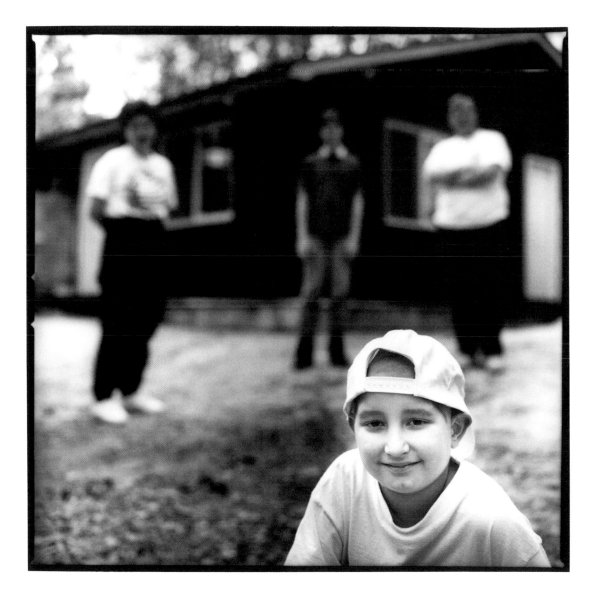

49

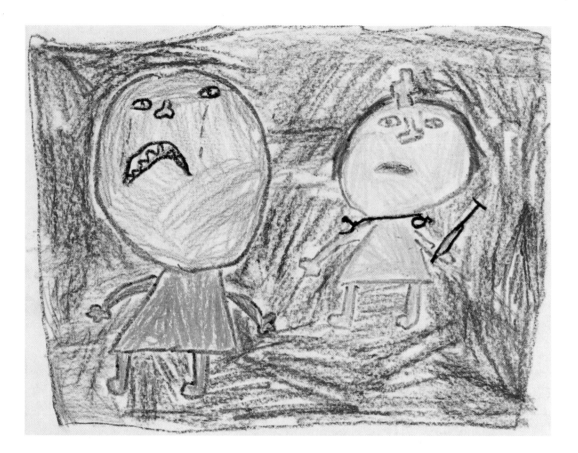

I have to get shots in my arm and my leg because I have leukemia.
It will make me better but sometimes I cry. Sometimes I don't.
It's okay that my hair is gone. It will grow back.

Helena
age 7

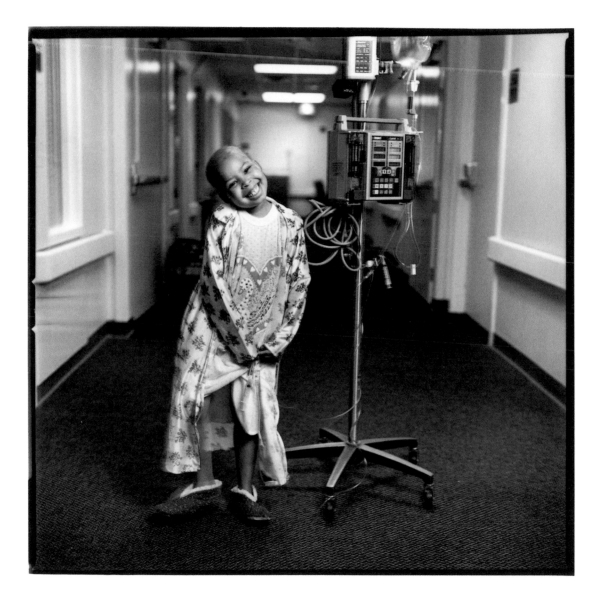

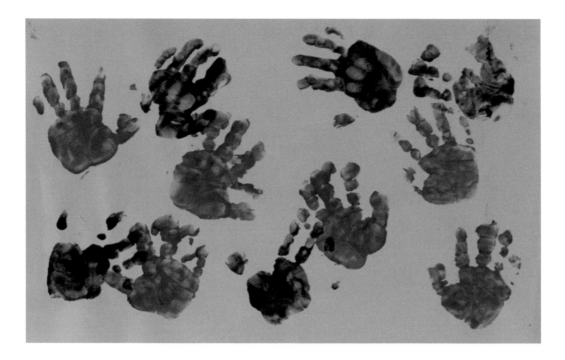

At six months of age, Meghan Head was diagnosed with acute lympho-
cytic leukemia with a lymphone component. After six months of
chemotherapy, she underwent a bone marrow transplant in January
1994. Her twin sister, Rachel, was her donor. Because Meghan and
Rachel are fraternal twins, there was only a 25 percent chance that
their bone marrow would be compatible. When the results from their
HLA typing showed their marrows identical, their father's response
was, "They truly are a match made in heaven."

Meghan
age 13 months

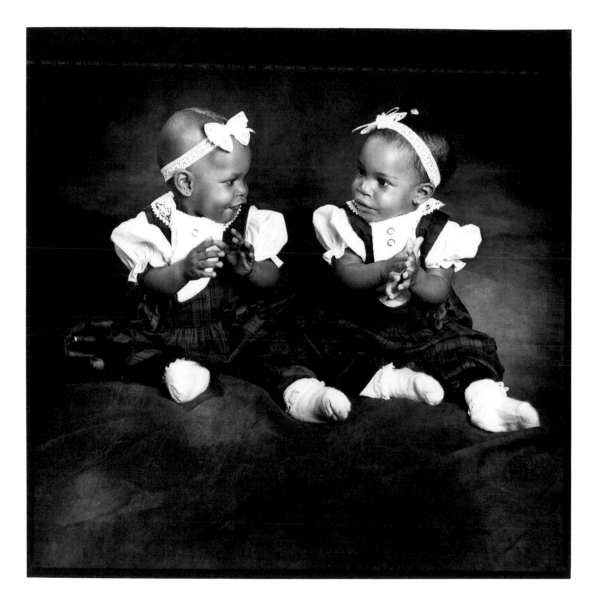

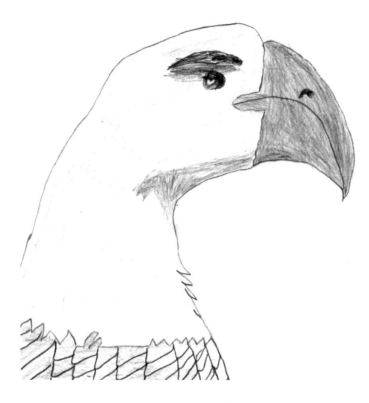

But they that wait upon the Lord shall renew their strength;
they shall mount up with wings as eagles; they shall run,
and not be weary; and they shall walk, not faint.

ISAIAH 40:31

David H.
age 8

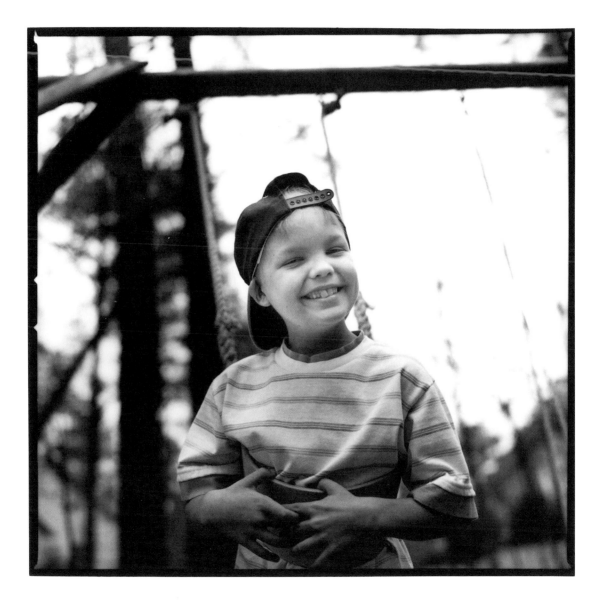

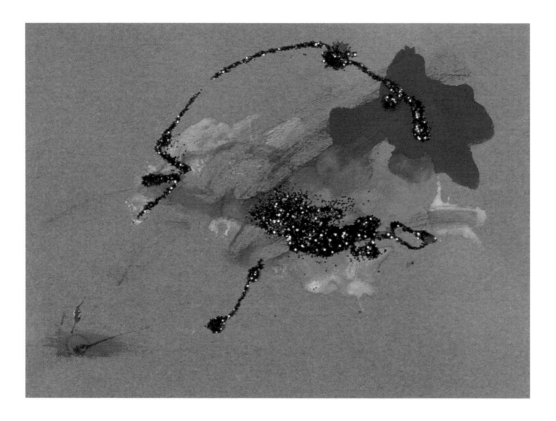

This is a picture of Ian Galloway Horner and Daddy
Galloway Horner and Annie Galloway Horner and
Mommy Galloway Horner.

Ian
age 3

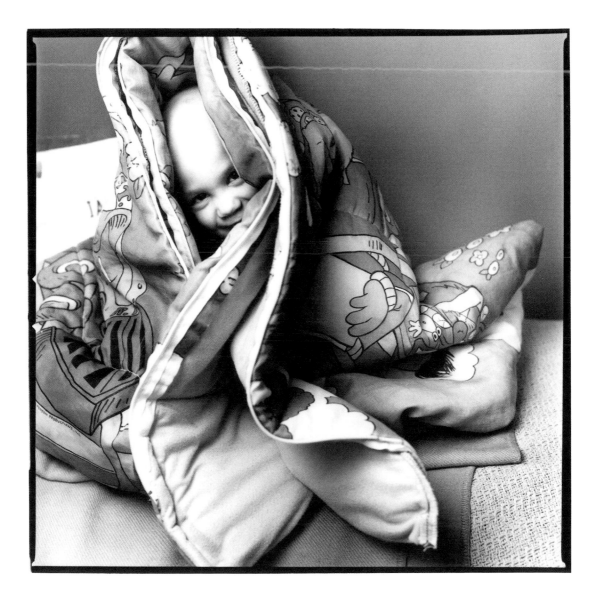

nobody had any advices

for the crisis   that was to come

I remember all the devices around my bed

yellow and clear bags over my head

sick and scared, losing hair

who said life isn't fair?

they sure said it

never know where our lives are headed

I take off my hat to any patient that relapsed

you're stronger than me

I could never go back

for to go through that again I'd rather leave

no more hospitals

out of sight, out of mind

I'd rather forget 'em

I can't be blamed for trying

this is how I explain the pain

instead of crying

MARCUS BRYANT, 2002

age 23

About us now

Eight years later . . .

seventeen of the children in this book survive. Billy Howard and Lisa Murray recently talked with them again and found they were engaged in many pursuits. One, the youngest, is in elementary school, but most are now in middle school, high school, or college. Four have completed their schooling and are pursuing careers, and two now have children of their own. Here is a brief look at their lives.

Eight years after she was treated for cancer, Amanda is twenty-two years of age, married to Craig, and has two children. Her son, Carter, is three years old, and her daughter, Mattie, is one.

Artavius, who eight years ago stood on his hospital bed and flexed his muscles for photographer Howard, is thirteen. As sometimes happens, chemotherapy left Artavius with medical problems. He has undergone a bone marrow transplant, and, most recently, a lung transplant, from which he is now recovering.

Barbara, who underwent cancer treatment at age fifteen, is now twenty-three and a senior at North Georgia College and State University. Barbara has been studying biology and would like to attend medical school.

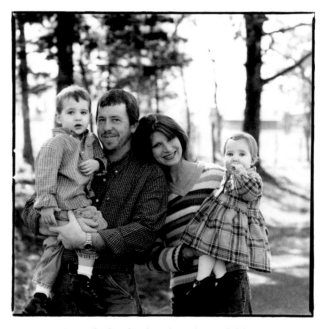

Amanda, her husband, and two children

Eight years ago, when Eric D. was ten, he drew a sandy beach and a deep blue ocean. He imagined he was there, he said, far from the problems of illness. Now Eric is eighteen, and a freshman at Macon College studying information technology.

Eric L., who was treated for cancer at age eleven, is now nineteen. He graduated from high school in the spring of 2002 and is an accomplished poet, his work having won awards in both local and nationwide contests. Like Artavius, Eric has had medical problems as a result of chemotherapy and underwent a heart transplant in 2001.

Helena, who eight years ago struck a jaunty pose with her rolling IV for photographer Howard, is now fifteen, and a freshman in high school.

Jared, who eight years ago drew Godzilla® attacking cancer, is now thirteen and in the eighth grade. He is involved in the performing arts, playing both piano and cello and trying his hand at acting.

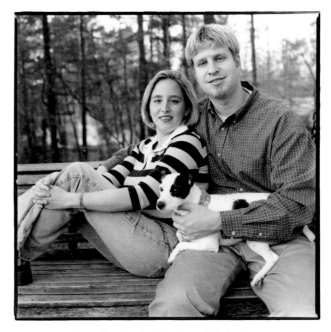

Jennifer, her husband, and their dog

Jennifer was eighteen when Howard photographed her and when she told Murray, "Having cancer has given me a new perspective on life. My views, goals, and beliefs have all changed. I am a much stronger and more profound person now." Jennifer is twenty-six. She is married to Zack and works as an insurance data analyst. Zack and Jennifer have a dog whose name is Adia.

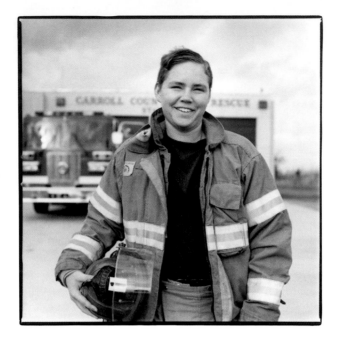

Jeremiah

When Jeremiah was thirteen, he drew a desert scene and told Murray, "Having cancer is like being all alone and lost in the desert." Today Jeremiah is twenty-one, and he has chosen a helping profession. He is a fireman and emergency medical technician.

Jessica B. was seven when she was being treated for cancer. A year later and in remission, she told Murray, "Now I'm at the end of my rainbow with the pot of gold. Now I'm just like everyone else." Jessica is fifteen, a freshman in high school, and in the National Honor Society.

Eight years ago, when Jessica S. was eleven, she lost her leg to cancer. Yet that same year, she was able to say to Murray, "Having my friends makes me want to keep on going. Friends are forever." "She discovered that life is all about connections," Howard said.

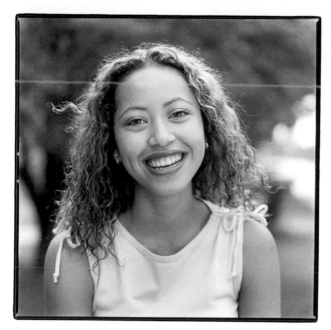

Kimsy

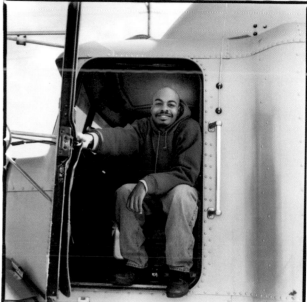

Marcus

"That is so powerful and so hard to learn." Now, at nineteen, she is a sophomore at Jacksonville State University in Jacksonville, Alabama, studying psychology.

Kelli, who relied heavily on her religious faith as she was being treated for cancer, is now twenty-one and about to graduate from Gainesville College in Gainesville, Georgia, with a degree in early childhood education. She plans to be married in the late summer of 2002.

Kimsy is now twenty-two. Daily, she makes her way around the Atlanta airport, working in various capacities to help provide security for Delta Airlines.

Marcus, now twenty-three, writes poetry and is enrolled in truck-driving school for "big rigs." His classmates, amazed at his sunny disposition, have nicknamed him "Smiley."

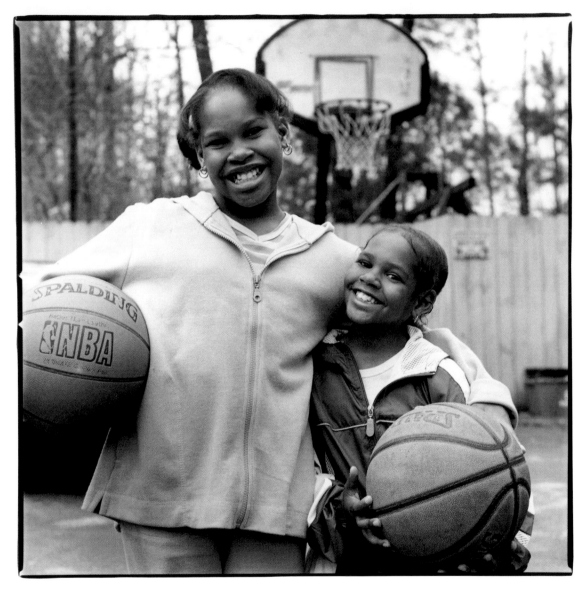

Rachel and Meghan

Meghan was only six months old when she began cancer treatment. Now she and her twin sister, Rachel, are nine and in the third grade, and both are standouts in basketball.

At age eight, Seth, sick and miserable from chemotherapy, pushed photographer Howard into a bank of sticker bushes. Both laughed about it and became friends. Now Seth is sixteen and a sophomore in high school. He no longer lunges at photographers and is said to be the recipient of many notes and phone calls from admiring female classmates.

Tonkya was eighteen when she underwent treatment for cancer. Now she cares for her four-year-old son, Donovan, during the day and goes to school at night. She is studying early childhood development.

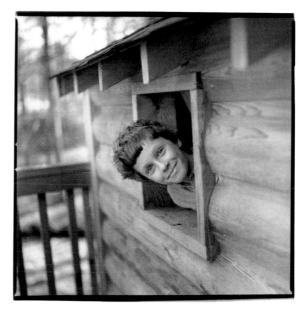

Seth, off therapy at age 7

Jacob's star

The courage and steadfast love of the children who did not survive cancer live on in the memories of those who knew them. One of those children was Jacob, who at the completion of his treatment in 1994 was glad to go home. Jacob had been five when he was first admitted to the hospital.

When Lisa Murray visited him in 1995, he was eager to show her that he was again a "regular kid" who could play outside without fear and who had a dog and a new baby brother. That summer day he drew another picture

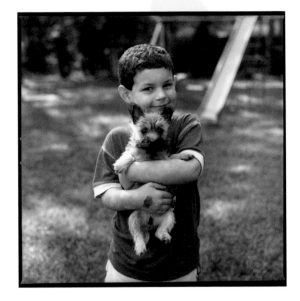

for her, this time showing a green and blue Earth set in the night sky. Beside Earth were stars and the moon, which he gave a smiling face. "Here's the man in the moon," he said. Jacob was happy.

But shortly after Murray's visit, Jacob's cancer returned. He went back to the hospital, and a year later, cancer claimed his life. Perhaps even as he sat with Murray and drew Earth as seen from far away, he had known in some deep part of himself that he would soon take his own place among the stars.

Now the night sky holds especial significance for Jacob's mother and the little brother of whom he was so proud. Often they leave the house on clear nights and search the sky until they find the bright light they have named "Jacob's star."

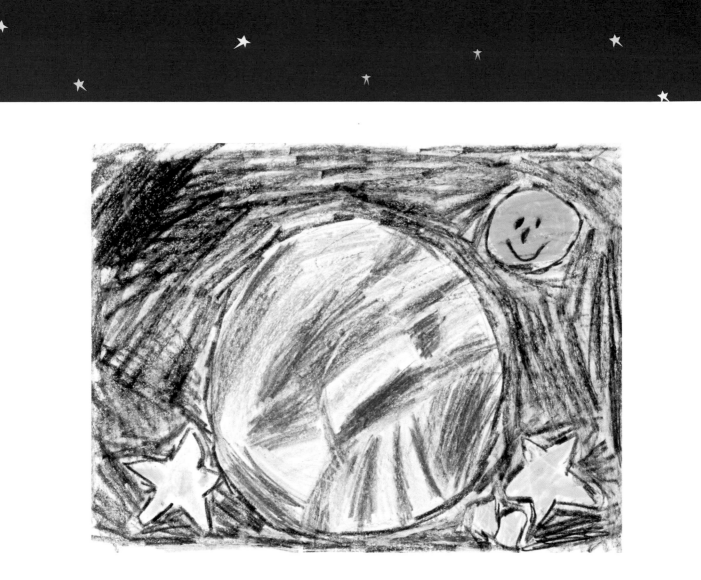

I'm free to the world now.
I can go outside and run and jump.
I feel great!

Information and resources

About the children	Age	Childhood cancer
Amanda	14	Osteogenic sarcoma
Artavius	6	Acute lymphocytic leukemia
Barbara	15	Large cell lymphoma
Courtney	9	Rhabdomyosarcoma
David H.	8	Acute lymphocytic leukemia
David T.	17	Osteogenic sarcoma
Eric D.	10	Neuroectodermal tumor
Eric L.	11	Osteogenic sarcoma
Grace	3	Neuroblastoma
Helena	7	Acute lymphocytic leukemia
Ian	3	Neuroblastoma
Jacob	5	Acute myelocytic leukemia
James	16	Acute lymphocytic leukemia
Jared	5	Burkitt's lymphoma
Jennifer	18	Large cell lymphoma
Jeremiah	13	Acute lymphocytic leukemia
Jessica B.	7	Rhabdomyosarcoma
Jessica S.	11	Osteogenic sarcoma
Katie	14	Synovial cell carcinoma
Kelli	13	Osteogenic sarcoma
Kimsy	14	Acute lymphocytic leukemia
Marcus	15	Acute lymphocytic leukemia
Meghan	13 months	Acute lymphocytic leukemia
Seth	8	Rhabdomyosarcoma
Tonkya	18	Osteogenic sarcoma

Resources
American Cancer Society

The American Cancer Society (ACS) provides educational materials and information on cancer, offers a variety of patient programs, and directs people to services in their community. To find your local office, contact us at 800-ACS-2345 or visit our web site (*http://www.cancer.org*).

Other Organizations

The following listings represent national organizations that provide some type of service or resource for children with cancer and their families. This list is designed to give you a starting point for seeking information, support, and needed resources. If you have a question that cannot be answered by one of the sources listed here, many of these organizations provide referrals, and your questions may be directed to other organizations or individuals.

Most of the organizations listed here can be contacted via phone, fax, mail, or e-mail, and some through their web site. Many of the web sites provide much of the same information that is available by postal mail. Keep in mind that new web sites appear daily while old ones expand, move, or disappear entirely. Some of the web sites or content outlined below may change. Often, a simple Internet search will point you to the new web site for a given organization. The ACS web site (*http://www.cancer.org*) provides links to other sources of cancer information and more.

The ACS does not endorse the agencies, organizations, corporations, and publications listed in this resource guide. This guide is provided for assistance in obtaining information only.

Pediatric Health and Cancer Organizations

American Academy of Pediatrics (AAP)

National Headquarters
141 Northwest Point Boulevard
Elk Grove Village, IL 60007-1098
Phone: 847-434-4000
Fax: 847-434-8000
Web site: *http://www.aap.org*

AAP is a member-based organization of pediatricians dedicated to the health, safety, and well-being of infants, children, adolescents, and young adults. The web site provides guidelines for pediatric cancer centers, related oncology links, and general information about childhood health.

American Pediatric Surgical Association (APSA)

60 Revere Drive, Suite 500
Northbrook, IL 60062
Phone: 847-480-9576
Fax: 847-480-9282
Web site: *http://www.eapsa.org*

The APSA is a surgical specialty organization composed of individuals who have dedicated themselves to the care of the pediatric surgical patient. The web site has a search feature to find a qualified pediatric surgeon (who is also a member of APSA) in your area.

American Society of Pediatric Hematology/Oncology (ASPH/O)

4700 West Lake
Glenview, IL 60025-1485
Phone: 847-375-4716
Fax: 847-375-6316
Web site: *http://www.aspho.org*

ASPH/O is a professional society of pediatric hematologists/oncologists who study and treat childhood cancer and blood diseases. The web site serves patients and families by providing a source of current peer-reviewed scientific and clinical research and links to find related information on the Internet.

Association of Pediatric Oncology Nurses (APON)

4700 West Lake Avenue
Glenview, IL 60025-1485
Phone: 847-375-4724
Fax: 847-734-8755
Web site: *http://www.apon.org*

APON is the professional organization for pediatric oncology nurses and other pediatric hematology/oncology health care professionals. Its members are dedicated to promoting optimal nursing care for children and adolescents with cancer and their families. Nurses who specialize in working with pediatric cancer patients may have passed an exam given by the APON to earn the designation of Certified Pediatric Oncology Nurse (CPON).

CancerSourceKids.com

Web site: *http://www.cancersourcekids.com*

Created by APON, the mission of CancerSourceKids.com is to be a secure site where children can learn about cancer in an interactive manner. It provides cancer information, games, and coping strategies for children and teens who have cancer and children and teens who have a sibling with cancer.

Brain Tumor Foundation for Children, Inc. (BTFC)

1835 Savoy Drive, Suite 316
Atlanta, GA 30341
Phone: 770-458-5554

Fax: 770-458-5467
Web site: *http://www.btfcgainc.org*

BTFC is a nonprofit organization whose members are friends, associates, and parents of children with brain tumors. BTFC provides information and emotional support to families of children with brain tumors, promotes public education and awareness of the disease, and raises funds to support research for a cure and for improvement in the treatment and the quality of life of children with brain tumors.

Childhood Brain Tumor Foundation (CBTF)

20312 Watkins Meadow Drive
Germantown, MD 20876
Toll-free: 877-217-4166
Phone: 301-515-2900
Web site: *http://www.childhoodbraintumor.org*

CBTF is a nonprofit organization founded by families, friends, and physicians of children with brain tumors. Their mission is to raise funds for scientific research, heighten public awareness, and improve prognosis and quality of life for those who are affected. The web site contains articles and newsletters about childhood brain tumors and information on the organization and its services.

Children's Brain Tumor Foundation (CBTF)

274 Madison Ave, Suite 1301
New York, NY 10016
Toll-free: 866-228-HOPE (866-228-4673)
Phone: 212-448-9494
Fax: 212-448-1022
Web site: *http://www.cbtf.org*

CBTF is a nonprofit organization whose mission is to improve the treatment, quality of life, and long-term outlook for children with brain and spinal cord tumors through research, support, education, and advocacy to families and survivors. CBTF provides:

- *A Resource Guide for Parents of Children With Brain or Spinal Cord Tumors*, a free publication that has information on the complexities of medical procedures, interruptions in school and social life, and uncertainty about the future
- Family Outreach Project, a joint program with Cancer Care, Inc., that provides support services for families and survivors of childhood brain tumors
- Parent-to-Parent Network, which puts experienced parents who want to share their knowledge and experiences in touch with parents in need
- Cosponsorship of conferences and seminars for families, survivors, and health care professionals, offering the latest information about research, treatments, and strategies for living
- Funding for research

The Children's Cause

1010 Wayne Avenue, Suite 770
Silver Spring, MD 20910
Phone: 301-562-2765
Fax: 301-565-9670
Web site: *http://www.childrenscause.org*

The Children's Cause is dedicated to accelerating the discovery of and access to innovative, safer, and more effective treatments for childhood cancer through education and advocacy. The web site provides information about FDA guidelines, NCI cancer policies, medical privacy issues, current clinical trials, and key resources.

Children's Leukemia Research Association (CLRA)

585 Stewart Avenue, Suite 18
Garden City, NY 11530
Phone: 516-222-1944 (may call collect)
Fax: 516-222-0457
Web site: *http://www.childrensleukemia.org*

CLRA is a nonprofit organization dedicated to raising funds to support efforts toward finding the causes and cures for leukemia. CLRA provides financial aid for treatment, medications, and lab fees for leukemia patients, public and professional education, and research grants to medical professionals.

Children's Oncology Group (COG)

P.O. Box 60012
Arcadia, CA 91066-6012
Toll-free: 800-458-6223
Phone: 626-447-0064
Fax: 626-445-4334
Web site: *http://www.childrensoncologygroup.org* or *http://www.conquerkidscancer.org*

COG is an NCI-supported clinical trials cooperative group devoted exclusively to childhood and adolescent cancer research. COG develops and coordinates cancer clinical trials. Their web site provides information about how to find a clinical trial for children with cancer. To find a member institution, call ACS at 800-ACS-2345.

Hope Street Kids

1600 Duke Street, Suite 110
Alexandria, VA 22314
Toll-free: 800-227-CRFA (800-227-2732)
Phone: 703-836-4412
Fax: 703-836-4413
Web site: *http://www.hopestreetkids.org*

Hope Street Kids is a children's initiative of the Cancer Research Foundation of America. The mission of Hope Street Kids is to eliminate childhood cancer through advocacy, education, and research and to support children with cancer and their families during and after treatment. Hope Street Kids assists both public and private research efforts through fundraising and provides leadership in advocating new research studies. The organization also translates the latest scientific breakthroughs into effective treatment and prevention strategies to improve the quality of life for all children.

Neuroblastoma Children's Cancer Society (NCCS)

P.O. Box 957672
Hoffman Estates, IL 60195
Toll-free: 800-532-5162
Fax: 847-490-0705
Web site: *http://www.neuroblastomacancer.org*

NCCS is a group of volunteers, many of whom have children or relatives who have, or have had, neuroblastoma. This organization is an advocate for children with neuroblastoma and is dedicated to serving as a support center for their families. The primary focus of NCCS is to raise money to assist local research in neuroblastoma cancer and to raise national awareness of the need for additional research and funding until a cure can be found.

Resources for Children with Cancer

American Cancer Society (ACS) Cancer Camps

Toll-free: 800-ACS-2345
Web site: http://www.cancer.org

In some areas, the Society sponsors camps for children who have, or have had, cancer. These camps are equipped to handle the special needs of children undergoing treatment. ACS divisions sponsor childhood cancer camps in more than 30 states. Please contact your local ACS office for a camp in your area. Individual camps will have more information about specific dates for the camp sessions.

Angel Locks, Inc.

P.O. Box 7116
North Arlington, NJ 07031
Toll-free: 877-93-LOCKS (877-935-6257)
Phone: 201-246-7979
Fax: 201-246-7970
Web site: *http://www.angellocks.org*

Angel Locks, Inc. is a nonprofit organization that provides quality, synthetic wigs to children with financial need who suffer from hair loss. The organization provides wigs to children up to age 18 who have hair loss due to, but not limited to, chemotherapy, leukemia, alopecia, and burns.

Childhood Leukemia Foundation (CLF)

1608 Route 88 West, Suite 203
Brick, NJ 08724
Toll-free: 888-CLF-7109 (888-253-7109)
Fax: 732-840-5818
Web site: *http://www.clf4kids.com*

CLF is a national nonprofit organization that nurtures the spirit of children with cancer. The web site provides general information about CLF and its services.

Children's Oncology Camping Association International (COCA)

Toll-free: 800-737-2667
Web site: *http://www.coca-intl.org*

COCA is an international assembly of people and member camps providing camping programs for children with cancer. For more information about their camps, visit the web site.

Give Kids the World Village

210 South Bass Road
Kissimmee, FL 34746
Toll-free: 800-995-KIDS (800-995-5437) for information on wish-granting foundations closest to the patient and their family
Phone: 407-396-1114
Fax: 407-396-1207
Web site: *http://www.gktw.org*

Give Kids the World Village is a nonprofit resort in Central Florida. It offers children with life-threatening illnesses the opportunity to experience the area's various theme parks. Families must be referred by one of the wish-granting organizations. Children ages 3–18, battling a life-threatening illness as deemed by a medical doctor, are eligible regardless of income. Information on wish fulfillment organizations that partner with Give Kids the World can be obtained by phone or on their web site.

Wigs for Kids

Executive Club Building
21330 Center Ridge Road, Suite C
Rocky River, OH 44116
Phone: 440-333-4433
Fax: 440-333-0200
Web site: *http://www.wigsforkids.org*

Wigs for Kids is a nonprofit organization providing hair replacement solutions for children affected by hair loss due to chemotherapy, radiation therapy, alopecia, burns, or other medical conditions.

Resources for Families with Children Who Have Cancer

AirLifeLine

50 Fullerton Court, Suite 200
Sacramento, CA 95825
Toll-free: 877-AIR-LIFE (877-247-5433)
Phone: 916-641-7800
Fax: 916-641-0600
Web site: *http://www.airlifeline.org*

AirLifeLine is a national nonprofit charitable organization of private pilots who fly ambulatory patients who cannot afford transportation to medical facilities for diagnosis and treatment. There is no charge for patients who qualify, and pilots can fly short or long trips, with distances as short as 50 miles. A support person may accompany the patient; however, AirLifeLine does not provide medical equipment or medical personnel. AirLifeLine and the ACS formed a partnership with the goal of making people across the United States aware of this transportation service.

Candlelighters Childhood Cancer Foundation (CCCF)

P.O. Box 498
Kensington, MD 20895-0498
Toll-free: 800-366-CCCF (800-366-2223)
Phone: 301-962-3520
Fax: 301-962-3521
Web site: *http://www.candlelighters.org*

CCCF is a national nonprofit organization whose mission is to educate, support, serve, and advocate for families of children with cancer, survivors of childhood cancer, and the health care professionals who care for them. The CCCF web site has information for families with newly diagnosed children, free publications, advocacy efforts, and inspirational links.

Children's Hospice International (CHI)

901 North Pitt Street, Suite 230
Alexandria, VA 22314
Toll-free: 800-2-4-CHILD (800-242-4453)
Phone: 703-684-0330
Fax: 703-684-0226
Web site: http://www.chionline.org

CHI is a nonprofit membership organization that provides a network of support to children with life-threatening conditions and their families. Through referral and information services, CHI facilitates the inclusion of children in existing and developing hospice and home care programs.

Compassionate Friends

National Headquarters
P.O. Box 3696
Oakbrook, IL 60522-3696
Toll-free: 877-969-0010
Phone: 630-990-0010
Fax: 630-990-0246
Web site: http://www.compassionatefriends.org

Compassionate Friends is a nationwide self-help organization offering support to families who have experienced the death of a child of any age, from any cause. It publishes a newsletter and other materials on parent and sibling bereavement. It makes referrals to nearly 600 local chapters.

Leukemia & Lymphoma Society

1311 Mamaroneck Avenue
White Plains, NY 10605
Toll-free: 800-955-4572 (Information Resource Center)
Phone: 914-949-5213
Fax: 914-949-6691
Web site: http://www.leukemia-lymphoma.org

Formerly known as the Leukemia Society of America (LSA), the Leukemia & Lymphoma Society is a national voluntary health agency dedicated to curing leukemia, lymphoma, Hodgkin's disease, and myeloma and to improving the quality of life of patients and their families. Patient service programs and resources include financial assistance, a telephone-based peer support network for newly diagnosed patients and family members, patient education and information, referral to local community resources and local chapters, and support groups. The web site has more information about their programs and services.

National Cancer Institute (NCI)

Pediatric Oncology Branch
Building 10, Room 13N240
Bethesda, MD 20892-1928
Toll-free: 800-624-4874
Phone: 301-496-4256
Fax: 301-401-0575
Web site: http://www-dcs.nci.nih.gov/pedonc

The Pediatric Oncology Branch of NCI has over two dozen active clinical trials, or treatment protocols, for a wide variety of childhood cancers. This branch has a 22-bed inpatient unit and extensive outpatient services. Children with newly diagnosed or recurrent cancer may be eligible for treatments. The web site provides information on the Pediatric Oncology Branch and its services.

National Children's Cancer Society (NCCS)

1015 Locust, Suite 600
St. Louis, MO 63101
Toll-free: 800-532-6459
Phone: 314-241-1600
Fax: 314-241-6949 (Program Services)
Web site: http://www.children-cancer.com

NCCS is a nonprofit national organization that helps children with cancer (newborns to age 18) and their families by providing support for their medical and emotional needs. The organization assists financially (including costs related to medical treatment such as lodging, meals, household needs, and travel) and provides advocacy, support services, education about childhood cancer as well as nutrition and tobacco information for children, and emotional support.

Operation Liftoff, Inc.

4204 Bonfils
Bridgeton, MO 63044
Phone: 314-298-9770
Fax: 314-298-1699
Web site: http://www.operationliftoff.com

Operation Liftoff is a nonprofit volunteer organization dedicated to providing trips within the United States for children 18 years of age and younger with life-threatening illnesses. When specialized treatment is required from medical specialists at health facilities distant from the home of a child, Operation Liftoff provides air travel for any qualifying child and both parents.

Ronald McDonald House Charities (RMHC)

McDonald's Corporation
One Kroc Drive, Department 014
Oak Brook, IL 60523
Phone: 630-623-7048 (charity information and donations)
Fax: 630-623-7488
Web site: http://www.rmhc.org

RMHC provides information about local Ronald McDonald Houses on a national and international basis. The Houses provide lodging for families of seriously ill children being treated away from home. The lodging is usually close to a hospital. The web site has a feature that locates a Ronald McDonald House in a specific area.

Wish Fulfillment Organizations

Many organizations grant wishes to chronically, seriously, or terminally ill children and adolescents. These organizations do not address medical or family financial needs, but they provide experiences that give respite to a child and family and fulfill wishes that a family may not be able to afford. Each organization has its own criteria for selection. If you are interested in such a program, you should check to see if your child meets the eligibility requirements and if the program has the services that you desire.

Bear Necessities Pediatric Cancer Foundation

85 West Algonquin Road, Suite 165
Arlington Heights, IL 60005
Phone: 847-952-9164
Fax: 847-952-0769
Web site: *http://www.bearnecessities.org*

Bear Necessities is a national organization dedicated to the fight against cancer by improving the quality of life for pediatric cancer patients and their families while furthering advancements in research. The Small Miracle program grants wishes for children with cancer so that they can forget their illness and enjoy being a child, if even for a moment.

Children's Hopes and Dreams Foundation

280 Route 46
Dover, NJ 07801
Phone: 973-361-7366
Fax: 908-459-9399
Web site: *http://www.childrenswishes.org*

Children's Hopes and Dreams Foundation is a nonprofit organization that serves chronically ill children between the ages of 4 and 17. The foundation also offers the Pen Pal Program, which matches ill children with other children diagnosed with chronic or life-threatening diseases or disabilities. To participate, call the organization for a free enrollment card.

Grant-A-Wish/The Children's Promise Foundation (Grant-A-Wish)

P.O. Box 21211
Baltimore, MD 21228
Toll-free: 800-933-5470
Web site: *http://www.grant-a-wish.org*

Grant-A-Wish is a national children's charity that provides supportive services to children 17 years old and younger who are battling life-threatening illnesses. This charity offers various programs that provide comfort and hope to these children.

Make-A-Wish Foundation of America

3550 North Central Avenue, Suite 300
Phoenix, AZ 85012-2127
Toll-free: 800-722-WISH (800-722-9474)
Phone: 602-279-WISH (602-279-9474)
Fax: 602-279-0855
Web site: *http://www.wish.org*

The Make-A-Wish Foundation grants the wishes of children with life-threatening illnesses. The web site has information about their program and eligibility requirements.

STARBRIGHT Foundation

11835 West Olympic Boulevard, Suite 500
Los Angeles, CA 90064
Phone: 310-479-1212
Fax: 310-479-1235
Web site: *http://www.starbright.org*

The STARBRIGHT Foundation is a nonprofit organization chaired by Steven Spielberg and General H. Norman Schwarzkopf. It is dedicated to the development of projects that empower seriously ill children to combat their medical and emotional challenges. STARBRIGHT projects address core issues that accompany illness—the pain, fear, loneliness, and depression that can be as damaging as the sickness itself. For more information on STARBRIGHT's programs, visit the web site.

Starlight Children's Foundation

5900 Wilshire Boulevard, Suite 2530
Los Angeles, CA 90036
Toll-free: 800-274-7827
Phone: 323-634-0080
Web site: *http://www.starlight.org*

Starlight Children's Foundation is an international nonprofit organization dedicated to improving the quality of life for seriously ill children 4–18 years old and their families. Information about Starlight programs is available on the web site.

The Sunshine Foundation

Corporate Office
1041 Mill Creek Drive
Feasterville, PA 19053
Toll-free: 800-767-1976
Phone: 215-396-4770
Fax: 215-396-4774
Web site: *http://www.sunshinefoundation.org*

The Sunshine Foundation is a nonprofit organization that serves children ages 3–21 years who are seriously ill, physically challenged, or abused. Sunshine's mission is to answer the dreams and wishes of these children.

Free Pamphlets and Booklets

American Brain Tumor Association. *A Primer of Brain Tumors, Seventh Edition: A Patient's Reference Manual.* Call 800-886-2282 for a free copy or view it online at *http://www.abta.org*.

American Brain Tumor Association. *When Your Child Is Ready to Return to School.* Call 800-886-2282 to order a free copy.

American Cancer Society. *After Diagnosis: A Guide for Patients and Families.* Booklet; Code #9440. Call 800-ACS-2345 (800-227-2345) for a free copy.

American Cancer Society. *Back to School: A Handbook for Parents of Children with Cancer.* Booklet; Code #4662. Call 800-ACS-2345 (800-227-2345) for a free copy.

American Cancer Society. *Closing the Umbrella.* Booklet; Code #2016. Call 800-ACS-2345 (800-227-2345) for a free copy.

American Cancer Society. *When Your Child Has Cancer.* Booklet; Code #4588. Call 800-ACS-2345 (800-227-2345) for a free copy.

Children's Brain Tumor Foundation. *A Resource Guide for Parents of Children With Brain or Spinal Cord Tumors.* Call 866-228-HOPE (866-228-4673) to obtain a free copy. Also available in Spanish.

Leukemia & Lymphoma Society. *Emotional Aspects of Childhood Leukemia: A Handbook for Parents.* Call 800-955-4572 for a free copy or view or order the handbook online at *http://www.leukemia-lymphoma.org*.

Leukemia & Lymphoma Society. *Understanding Chemotherapy.* Call 800-955-4572 for a free copy or view or order it online at *http://www.leukemia-lymphoma.org*.

National Cancer Institute. *Eating Hints for Cancer Patients.* 1997. NIH Publication No. 98-2079. Call 800-4-CANCER (800-422-6237) for a free copy or view it online at *http://www.cancer.gov* under Cancer Information.

National Cancer Institute. *Taking Part in Clinical Trials: What Cancer Patients Need to Know.* 1998. NIH Publication No. 97-4250. Call 800-4-CANCER (800-422-6237) for a free copy or view it online at *http://www.cancer.gov* under Cancer Information.

National Cancer Institute. *When Someone in Your Family Has Cancer.* 1990. Write to Publications Ordering Service, P.O. Box 24128, Baltimore, MD 21227, call 800-4-CANCER (800-422-6237), or view it online at *http://www.cancer.gov* under Cancer Information.

National Cancer Institute. *Young People with Cancer: A Handbook for Parents.* 1991. NIH Publication No. 01-2378. Call 800-4-CANCER (800-422-6237) for a free copy or view it online at *http://www.cancer.gov* under Cancer Information.

National Children's Cancer Society. *Book of Me.* Call 800-532-6459 for a free copy for your child or order it online at *http://www.children-cancer.com*.

Acknowledgments

Many people contributed to the making of this book. On top of the heap are the doctors, nurses, and staff of the oncology unit at Egleston Children's Hospital, now Children's Healthcare of Atlanta at Egleston, who cared for the bodies and spirits of all the children in these pages.

Before there was a book, there was an exhibition. Marcia Wood Gallery provided a space to display the children's art when it was first introduced, and Sally Wood at Toco Hill Picture Framing made the frames. The Woods are soldiers for beauty, and we are grateful for their support.

Funding for the art exhibition was generously provided by The Georgia Council for the Arts, CURE Childhood Cancer, and The Brain Tumor Foundation for Children, Incorporated.

Now, with the help of the American Cancer Society, the exhibition finds its way into print. Their belief in the message presented by the children has made this book possible.

Becky Lavender—social worker, miracle worker, and ace detective—helped track down the families of the twenty-five children, whom we had not seen in the eight years since the exhibition. Beth Bassett finessed the language into a beautiful pattern of words bringing to life the experience we both felt, and Pam Drake's magic eye captured our likenesses for the book.

Susan Walker has been a longstanding, enduring, consistent supporter for families and their children with cancer. Her commitment to them has its roots in personal experience. She lost her own child to this disease.

We thank Jeff Foxworthy, a very funny guy with a heart of gold, who for years has quietly volunteered his time, his humor, and his money for children with cancer. His work at Duke's Children's Hospital and Camp Sunshine has, according to him, given him much more than he could hope to give in return.

Finally, we thank Laurie Shock for encouraging us to publish this work and for donating her time to design a book that honors the children who have shared their lives with us.

— *Lisa Murray and Billy Howard*

About the authors

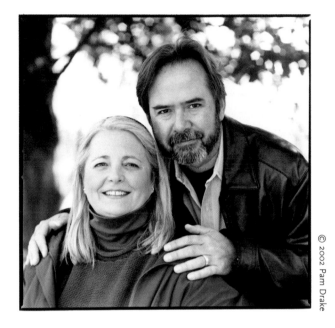

© 2002 Pam Drake

Lisa Murray is a Board-Certified and Registered Art Therapist with the American Art Therapy Association. She received her training at Emporia State University and interned at the Menninger Foundation in Topeka, Kansas. She has worked with children in hospitals for more than twenty years.

She lives in Stone Mountain, Georgia, with her husband, Lewis, and two sons, Clark and Joe.

Billy Howard is a commercial and documentary photographer with an emphasis on health, education, and social themes.

He is the author of *Epitaphs for the Living: Words and Images in the Time of AIDS* and *Portrait of Spirit: One Story at a Time*, images and interviews of people with disabilities, with a foreword by Christopher Reeve and interviews by Maggie Holtzberg.

He lives in Atlanta with his wife, Laurie, and their cat, Allie.

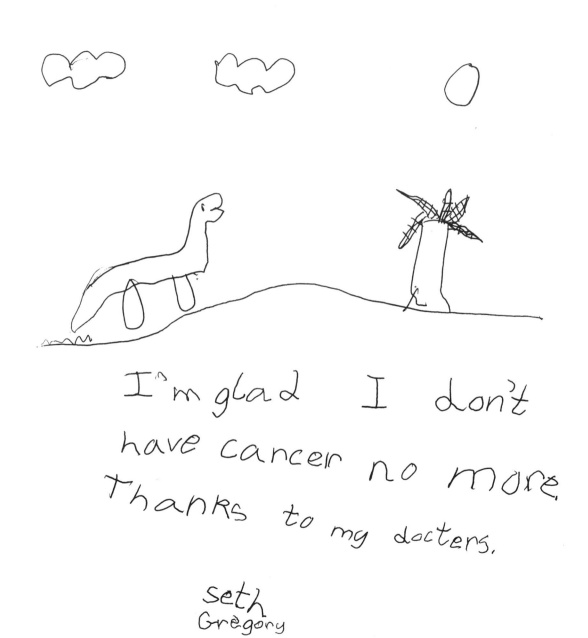

I'm glad I don't have cancer no more. Thanks to my docters.

seth
Gregory